# Gymsanity

## A humorous take on gym insanity

KEVA SILVERSMITH

-Overheard at the gym today: "I'm training harder than ever, man. I even came to the gym on my off day to go in the steam room."

# CONTENTS

# INTRODUCTION

Every fitness buff is familiar with the various yahoos that take up space at the gym. There are the folks who mean well but nevertheless exhibit terrible form. Then there are the people, less well intentioned, who simply put forth a lousy effort. Potentially worse than the lousy effort are those whose absurd approach to training creates a danger to themselves or others. None of this really impacts you, the serious lifter, until an individual's lack of etiquette, or the quality of the gym itself, interferes with your workout. Of course, some gym behavior, while not actually violating your space, creates such a spectacle that it still distracts from your workout. Here we go.

# 1 THE PEOPLE WHO MEAN WELL
# BUT EXHIBIT TERRIBLE FORM

**Perfect Form**

I had been pondering ways to increase the readership of my blog when a trip through a grocery store checkout line sparked an idea. If established fitness magazines could use this gimmick to boost circulation, then so could I. Flex Magazine put on its cover a young Arnold Schwarzenegger.

I've often thought about why Arnold continues to inspire fitness enthusiasts nearly three decades after his retirement from professional bodybuilding. He hasn't even appeared shirtless in a movie in any significant way since the early 1990's.

Arnold's main appeal can't be his size in his prime. Professional bodybuilders these days run thicker with better definition. Mr. Olympia 2014 stands 5'9" at 265 pounds, compared to Schwarzenegger's championship reign at 6'1", 245 pounds. Incidentally, this is no dig at Arnold. Today's gym equipment is better, the science of fitness is more advanced, and the … well … performance enhancers probably give you more bang for the buck.

In my opinion, the continued fascination with Arnold results from the classic, sweeping artistry of his physique. Many of Arnold's aesthetic gifts can, of course, be attributed to his good fortune with genetics. Take a look at his biceps. The typical bicep muscle terminates about an inch ahead of the forearm, while Arnold's bicep fills the entire space between his front shoulder and elbow. The same principle applies to Arnold's back. My lat muscle ties in around the middle of my rib cage. Arnold's wings taper off virtually at his waist.

But there's a second factor at work: Arnold was a perfectionist when it came to proper lifting form. Beyond genes, Arnold's long, graceful lines are the result of muscles worked in a controlled fashion through a full range of motion. His superior lifting technique lengthened his muscles and engaged the largest possible number of muscle fibers.

Walk into a gym today, however, and you'll find people performing all manner of abbreviated lifts: pull-ups that reach neither peak contraction at the top nor full extension at the bottom; overloaded squats that result in no serious bend in the knees; bicep preacher curls that stop a good 20 degrees short of straight arms. Excessive weight, laziness and all around bad habits have turned core lifts into a real live exercise in futility.

What was true in Arnold's day remains true today. Progress is not determined by how much weight you can move, but how much weight you can move with perfect form.

## Not So Perfect Form

A reader sent me a question about Arnold and the current state of bodybuilding:

> Have you seen the way Ronnie Coleman trains? He has the worst form I ever saw and yet he has won Mr. Olympia eight times. Personally I don't think modern bodybuilders look as good as Arnie did but you say "Professional bodybuilders these days run thicker with better definition," and Ronnie Coleman is I am sure exactly what you are talking about - 5'11" 285 lbs contest weight. Look up videos of him training on YouTube. His form is terrible. I used to believe in perfect form too but seeing Coleman train changed my opinion completely. I sometimes use heavy weight with bad form and find my muscles aching painfully the next day. Of course the painful muscles lead to growth. Any thoughts?

My response:

I checked out the Coleman videos as you suggested. There, just like you said: T-bar rows done standing ramrod straight, and some kind of bent over dumbbell row targeting neither lats nor rear delts. On the other hand, I had never seen before anyone do a perfect set of 10 bench presses with 200 pound dumbbells. And you have to admit, his knees did reach 90 degrees on his 2300 pound leg presses.

Arnold wrote in his bodybuilding encyclopedia that some genetic freaks can bulk up by just walking past a dumbbell rack. Coleman might be the most genetically gifted bodybuilder since Sergio Oliva - and be able to grow massively even with sloppy form. But just think of where he'd be if he did things right!

I can imagine that bad form creates all kinds of aches and pains for you. It's hard for me to say that this is "good" soreness, however, and not just muscles torn and twisted by improper technique.

There's probably something to be said for occasionally stressing your muscles with very heavy weight - a version of the Weider muscle confusion principle. And cheating to push your muscles to new gains is a part of every bodybuilder's repertoire. But without Ronnie Coleman's genes, I can't see that strategy forming the core of a successful fitness program.

## Heart Attack

Given the far-reaching ignorant and even reckless use of gym equipment, I write the following with a full understanding of its magnitude: No equipment in the gym falls victim to more mistakes, blunders and downright wasted motion than the poor cardio machines.

First, a simple tip. When you ride the stationary bike, always use the pedal straps. If you start wheeling around like a three-year-old on a tricycle, you deprive yourself of 50 percent of the workout – the stress on the hamstring that comes from the upstroke.

On the treadmill, keep your hands to yourself. Every day, I see hands locked to the top of dashboards, fingers wrapped around front handles, and hands gripping side rails. When you use your arms to pull yourself along, the solid workout that comes from even a simple brisk walk gets transferred to a bunch of rubber and plastic. Remember, until Skynet goes active, we still control the machines. If you can't survive your workout without clinging to the treadmill, lower the incline, reduce the speed.

Then there's the StairMaster. We've got riders draping themselves over the machine like an oversized towel; people inverting their grip – with elbows locked out - so feet barely touch pedals; folks engrossed in books, journals and all manner of periodicals propped up at eye level while supposedly "working out"; and people cranking machines to a speed that forces them to hang onto the stepper's front handles for dear life. Guys: head up, back straight, side rails used only for balance. I know it's hard. That's why it's called … exercise.

One last thing. If you're staring at a row of empty treadmills, don't climb onto the one exactly next to me. Put at least one machine between me and your coughing and sweating. This same rule also applies to seating in a movie theatre.[1]

## Hard Gainers

Although a certain segment of the population goes out of its way to avoid making progress in the gym (see Chapter 2), hard gainers – or "hardgainers" (an actual fitness term of art) – find their bodybuilding dreams limited by mediocre genetics. I've seen studies that estimate between 60 and 95 percent of people are hardgainers.

These figures aren't all that surprising. In any sport, a few elite athletes set the standard for legions of amateurs. And besides, statistically speaking, most people are average.

I, however, would like to advance a new theory. In my estimation, when it comes to building muscle, the problem is that 60 to 95 percent of people have no idea what they're doing.

Today at the gym I watched a couple younger guys make an absolute mess of their back workout. They performed sets of t-bar rows and barbell rows with their posture nearly ramrod straight, transforming these excellent mass builders into sloppy bicep curls.

Then there are the folks who turn a simple set of abdominal crunches into a chiropractor's nightmare. Lying on the floor, they wrap their arms tightly around their heads, and yank their chin into their upper chests over and over. I don't know which is more remarkable – the 30, even 50, reps per set performed this way, or the ability to spend this much energy on abs without tapping even one stomach muscle fiber. Either way, I urge you people, why don't you start by trying to execute just one clean crunch – fingers behind the ears, chin up, strong contraction in the abs. Just one.

---

[1] Sophia Vergara excepted.

## Seductively Simple

I'm not kidding when I say that folks struggling with good form should focus first on doing just one clean, quality rep. I can think of a number of bodyweight exercises where this rule applies: crunches, dips and certainly unassisted pull-ups.

Today at the gym, however, I saw another kind of one rep exercise that is most definitely not what I have in mind. It's the all too familiar group of guys who prepare for bench presses by loading a minivan onto each side of the barbell.

The terrible form, sure to follow, doesn't defeat just the philosophical purpose of my "one rep" rule. On a physiological level, the only possible benefit derived from singles is the strengthening of ligaments - an advantage clearly outweighed by the increased risk of injury. (And on a practical level, the spotter basically does a barbell row while the bencher just grunts a lot.) One rep max lifts grow very little muscle, contrary to the hopes of high school football players and frat boys. Just compare the muscularity between Olympic weightlifters and serious amateur bodybuilders.

Nevertheless, a discussion of muscle biology misses a far more interesting sociological point. These guys load up a bunch of weight so they can lean conspicuously against their barbell and grin idiotically when attractive women pass by.

In fact, I think there is an opportunity here to launch the next innovation in seduction techniques. Go ahead and load up your barbell - stand around - but don't actually lift at all. The most productive part of the max workout comes from the effort loading and unloading several 45 pound plates anyway. Why find yourself lying on the bench, wasting a few precious seconds, when the next 10 out of 10 walks by? Most importantly, why risk breaking a sweat?

There can be too much of a good thing, however. Just because one rep is too few doesn't mean that peak muscularity comes from doing 50. The muscle building sweet spot is somewhere between six and eight reps per set (for women, I'll call it the muscle *toning* sweet spot). Scientific studies also encourage a little variety in your workout: 6-8 reps to work the explosive "fast-twitch" muscle fibers, 10-12 reps to stimulate the endurance "slow-twitch" fibers.

Either way, you should be using a weight heavy enough that you experience muscle failure by the tenth, maybe twelfth rep. You're just cheating yourself on multiple levels if you pick a weight with which you can do 30, but simply stop at 10. Regardless, once you enter the 12-15 rep range and beyond, your workout becomes a form of endurance training, not muscle building.

Besides, if you can really do dozens of reps - particularly when it comes to abs – you're probably not doing the movement right at all.

## Low Back Special

I cheer new techniques and machines that target the low back. In fact, I just completed a month of physical therapy for a herniated disk, the consequence of fanatical free weight workouts during my early 20's.

One good alternative is the basic back extension machine. You sit in the machine, select the weight, and work your spinal erectors by leaning against the back pad. Sounds simple enough, right? Well, today I saw a woman raise the machine's adjustable back pad so that it lay directly across the top of her spine. By stiffening her neck and pressing back with her head, she managed to push the machine through its normal motion.

Still, no back exercise, done correctly or otherwise, is as dangerous as the good morning. A good morning consists of standing under a heavy barbell and bending forward at the waist, all while keeping your legs straight. This movement has fallen out of favor over time, either as a result of advances in kinesiology or its contribution to long lines at sports medicine clinics. I've even been to a gym that crossed out the good morning image on its poster of suggested back exercises.

I occasionally notice women doing this exercise with just a Body Bar, though I imagine the risk of injury at these weights is minimal. I did recently find a serious lifter mocking a gym novice online for not knowing the difference between squats and the good mornings the serious lifter was actually performing.

Well, pal, the joke's on you. My greatest regret as a trainer is the way I encouraged many clients to add good mornings to their workouts. Though I was only passing on the best information at the time, these folks are probably cursing me from the straps of a traction machine right now.

The deadlift, on the other hand, remains one of the sport's best overall strength and mass builders – as long as you pay meticulous attention to proper form. Here's an example I found on a training website of what not to do:

> There was a guy at my gym that worked out while his girlfriend did. He would "show off" on deadlift day for her. His idea of a deadlift was to drop to the floor at light speed, smash the plates off the floor, then bounce it up to the start position and call that a rep. He sounded like a grocery cart being pushed down the stairs.

The correct mechanical position for beginning and finishing the deadlift: head up, shoulders higher than butt, and your butt higher than knees. Also, it's important to feel yourself pushing with your legs rather than lifting with your back. I offer no guarantees, however, only the assurance that I'm passing on the best information available today.

### Top Two Dumbest Things I've Ever Seen at the Gym

I'll just cut to the chase. The second most absurd thing I have ever seen in the gym was a fellow running on the treadmill in flip-flops. This gentleman was not walking leisurely or warming up, but engaged in a full blown 30 minute run in his beach footwear.

Now #1: It's bad enough when members bring their cellphones onto the gym floor. You've got the distractions of phones ringing, silly conversations (and my favorite: dude with headphones on so he doesn't hear his own phone ringing). One guy resolved all these logistical problems by wearing his Bluetooth hands free headset onto the gym floor. The most amazing thing I have ever seen in a gym was this guy doing a set of 10-15 pull-ups *while talking on the phone*.

I took clarinet lessons when I was young, and my teacher held a yearly recital for all her students. One year, a saxophonist played through his entire concerto with gum in his mouth, sometimes chewing. Much like Bluetooth man, the performance was not remarkable for its quality, but for the ability to combine previously mutually exclusive activities.

# 2 THE PEOPLE WHO PUT FORTH
# A LOUSY EFFORT

## Save Me Some Bordeaux

I learned a great line out on the golf course recently. To the incredibly slow foursome ahead of us, a guy in my group yelled out "Save us some brie!" Get it? The foursome was moving at such a snail's pace it was like they were having a picnic out on the fairway.

At the gym, I come across similar folks who plop down on a piece of equipment like it's a leather couch at a dinner party. Today, I watched a guy take up residence on an incline Hammer Smith machine for about three-quarters of an hour. (This is not an exaggeration – there is a clock directly above the machine.) I'm sure it was quite relaxing: the back rest allows you to recline at a slight angle, the handle bars provide a great place to prop up your arms. He also received several visitors during his morning of leisure, where they considered the current issues of the day. Other than when he first sat down, this guy did not perform one set on the machine.

As I walked past the confab on my way to the locker room (I had completed my entire workout) I muttered, "Save me some Bordeaux."

## The Four-Legged Leg Press

Although I am frequently dismayed by people's laziness and all around carelessness in the gym (obviously: I've written a book about it), I am equally impressed by how creatively they accomplish nothing.

When it comes to training legs, people generally steer clear altogether. Squat racks, leg press machines and Smith machines collect the most dust in the gym, while people congregate around equipment that works the smaller muscle groups. And why not: training legs hurts like crap! Properly training the body's largest and strongest muscle group requires a serious commitment to intensity and concentration.

So let's talk about a way people train legs unseriously. I've noticed two distinct methods people use to cheat on the leg press. The first is when the guy does his set with his arms crossed over his chest, so that he severely limits the lift's range of motion. The second, and my favorite, is when the guy presses his hands to his knees throughout the lift. He cheats himself twice: On the eccentric (down) portion of the lift, he uses his upper body to help resist the weight of the carriage; during the concentric (up) part of the lift, he pushes like hell with his upper body to return the carriage back to its starting point.

In the extreme, this four-legged leg press becomes a veritable bench press, recruiting heavy involvement from the chest, shoulders and triceps. You might even be able to build some upper body strength this way. (I can hear my father's snark now: "Wouldn't this actually be a *more* efficient way to lift – to work all these body parts at once?!?") Well, it may in fact be more efficient, but it certainly isn't more effective.

## Going Out On a High Note

So here's one. I'm resting between sets of bench presses, and I notice a guy come in and drop his gym bag next to the squat rack. He throws three plates onto each side of the bar, warms up with a quick check of his nose hairs in the mirror, and then settles in for his lift. What luck: I am present for the setting of a new land speed record, 0-300 in about ten seconds flat.

My high school band teacher always insisted that the proper way to warm up is not to pick out the highest note you can play and blow it as long and loudly as you can. Likewise, a warm up in the gym needs to be a thoughtful process that maximizes strength while minimizing the risk of injury.

The specifics aren't critical; you've warmed up adequately when you're ready to hit your first heavy set at full weight. My father, in his home gym, first picks up all the ping pong balls so inconsiderately left on the floor from the night before. I warm up with a 3-5 minute stroll on the treadmill, followed by stretching combined with three light sets of the first lift I plan to perform.

And what happened with Minuteman over at the squat rack? No, he didn't tear a quad muscle or rip apart his knee. In fact, he didn't squat deep enough to do much of anything at all.

## Belt Buckle

Hang out in the grunting area of your gym, and you're destined to find folks using lifting belts and joint wraps to excess. I read somewhere that these guys who wrap their knees, their elbows, their wrists and then cinch a weight belt around their waists begin to resemble mummies. Bodybuilding forums debate at length whether these lifting aids improve safety, or whether they simply help stabilize the ego by increasing the amount of weight that a person can lift.

What's more interesting to me, however, are the guys who strap on a heavy-duty lifting belt as some kind of fashion statement. I've seen various levels of absurdity:

Stage 1) Belt on during bench presses. Seeing as you literally lie down on your back muscles during a bench press, the only reason to wear a belt is if you plan on violently arching your back in a frantic attempt to return the barbell to its starting point. This maneuver could be considered poor form.

Stage 2) Belt on during leg presses. This use of a belt is quite peculiar since you're sitting down with your entire upper body reclining on a thick pad. I can't imagine how a lifting belt does anything other than chafe against your hip flexors during the movement.

Stage 3) Now we're entering deep madness. I once saw a guy tighten his lifting belt before performing a set of seated calf raises.

Stage 4) This is where you stop and stare. There was a guy at the gym today with his lifting belt on riding the elliptical machine. Not only is the elliptical machine lower impact than plain walking, but let's face it: if your back is in such bad shape that you need a belt to remain upright, you should probably be in bed.

I considered following this guy into the locker room to see if he wore his belt in the shower too. But hey, I'm only willing to go so far for this blog.

## 24 Hour Fitness

One of the most underrated – underhyped – benefits of weight training is the 24/7 calorie furnace created by slabs of lean muscle. Much like the basketball player who's still 6'10" even when he's tired, your toned physique is burning fuel when you're on the couch watching TV, or even asleep.

Meaningful lean mass is achieved by developing the body's largest muscles (legs, back and chest) through exercises that, naturally, hurt the most. I'm referring to the moves that make a difference: squats, deadlifts, rowing movements, various kinds of presses.

Unfortunately, folks at the gym throw away daily this round-the-clock fitness opportunity. And of course, the worst offenders are usually the people who need it most. I see flabby middle-aged women wasting their time with moves like one-arm tricep pulldowns or concentration curls. I shake my head watching paunchy guys perform isolation exercises like pec-deck flys or leg extensions. All these movements should belong exclusively to serious bodybuilders, who are looking to bring out the striations in their already-meaty legs, pecs and arms.

The most depressing part is that these folks are often exercising under the close watch of personal trainers. People with limited time and limited goals should especially be directed toward major compound movements; key exercises like rows and presses work smaller muscle groups – shoulders, arms – at the same time.

One of these days I'm going to have to step in and give a free lesson myself.

## Lazy

I always get a kick out of watching big burly guys use the seated leg curl. Few people realize this machine was designed specifically for pregnant women (who can't lie on their stomach to perform a traditional hamstring curl). Still, the machine does a good job of targeting the hamstrings; it's a respectable alternative to the horizontal version.

I'm not nearly as positive about the stationary hand cycle. The hand cycle provides a cardiovascular option for wheelchair-bound athletes. The able-bodied person using the hand cycle has skipped the treadmill, the StairMaster, the elliptical machine, and of course, the stationary bike, in order to experience a workout that is literally handicapped.

I notice two kinds of laziness at the gym. There's typical sloth, and then there's why bother to show up at all. The woman sitting in the hand cycle today most definitely burned the bulk of her calories walking from the parking lot to the gym. It's one thing to choose a machine that uses only the body's smaller muscle groups when your focus ought to be maximizing calorie burn. It's quite another to rotate the crank so slowly that the fat hanging from your upper arms doesn't even jiggle.

No matter. I think it was excellent training for repeated lifting of her TV's remote control.

## Equipment Failure

There's an old law school joke about the failing student with a bookshelf full of books. Performing terribly, he doesn't crack the binding on the books he already owns, but instead goes out and buys more books.

At the gym yesterday, I noticed this scrawny guy with brilliant white running shoes striding into the leg area. The strap from his bulging gym bag cut into his shoulder. In one hand he clutched a sagging plastic grocery bag, while in the other he carried a full gallon jug of water. He also had a clipboard tucked under his arm that held a half-inch stack of papers.

I took a final swig from my own one pint water bottle and decided to grab a seat on a nearby machine. I knew we were about to see something special.

For nearly 10 minutes, this guy struggled to set the squat rack safeties to their highest position. He finally gave up and moved to the Smith Machine, pushing the bar to its highest setting and throwing a 45 pound plate on each side. With arms fully extended, he unracked the bar and held it steady for a few seconds, then let it drop back in place.

He sat down, grabbed his clipboard, and proceeded to take lengthy notes. Obviously, he needed a detailed record of this major progress.

## Whatever It Takes

A heavyset gentleman stepped onto the locker room scale. He looked down at the digits, then sighed in disgust and cursed loudly. He raised his head and glowered at the reflection in the mirror. His eyes betrayed his anger at himself, and then expressed a fresh resolve.

As he turned to leave, the guy nodded to an acquaintance passing by.

"See you tomorrow?" his friend asked.

"Naah," the guy responded. "Maybe Tuesday."

# 3 THE PEOPLE WHO CREATE A DANGER TO THEMSELVES OR OTHERS

## The One-Armed Spot

The typical bench press spot is bad enough: some egomaniac loads his barbell with far too much weight for him to handle, forcing the poor spotter to deadlift the barbell off the lifter's chest. What I saw yesterday, however, has to qualify as spotter's revenge. Turned sideways, with his hip nearly touching the lifter's head, this spotter reached out, grabbed the middle of the barbell, and proceeded to spot with one arm.

Now, the spotter's intent was not create an incredibly dangerous situation, where he has no leverage in the event of an emergency (while also increasing the risk that his arm gets torn off). He also did not plan to cause a serious imbalance for the lifter, with his tenuous grip pulling unevenly somewhere near the bar's mid-line. No, the spotter thought he looked like a real bad-ass, so powerful he can't even be bothered to spot with two hands. Like I said, spotter's revenge.

## Speaking Truth to Power

I know that golf is supposed to be the sport most metaphorically applicable to life. But I'd like to mention this bit of insight that came from my coach of youth soccer: A ball rolling slowly towards the goal has a much greater chance of scoring than a fast wild shot that is off the mark. This wisdom is clearly applicable to something like financial planning, and also to the gym.

I used to deadlift extremely heavy – my best sets were 335 pounds for six reps, with no belt on. I'm also proud to say that my form was perfect. However, the only way I could get out of a car for one week following was to open the door and roll out onto the ground.

Today, as I watched an average-sized guy load up a barbell with four plates on a side, my amusement was tempered by empathy.

For a regular guy, a 405 pound deadlift is preposterous. To be sure, I'd never before seen a person deadlift with a spotter, getting pulled upright at the top of each rep. I did, however, recognize the noise this guy made bouncing his barbell as a grocery cart being pushed down the stairs. Regardless, when this fellow added another 25 pound plate between sets, I didn't even bother to continue watching. I just turned away and waited for the sound of splintering low back ligaments.

Nowadays, I do my sets of deadlifts at about 225 pounds for eight or nine reps. I'm no longer the man to call to lift a car off some unfortunate soul, but I'm also not missing bunches of workouts due to a wrecked low back. I figure it's better to be at the gym making slow but regular progress, than to engage in one fast wild workout and spend the next several days in bed.

## A Parents' Guide to Working Out

I think parents of young children enter into the experience with some awareness of the expenditures that lie ahead. There's the monetary cost, obviously, and also the drain of intangibles: time, energy and peace. But what has been a surprise to me, at least, is the physical damage my kids inflict on me – and the resulting missed workouts at the gym.

For example, a couple years ago I took my son to a University of Michigan alumni event, where he could meet the head coaches of the football, basketball and hockey programs. In order for my son to see the guests of honor, I had to lift him onto my shoulders, where he sat comfortably for the 30 minute program. At the end of the event, my son got a football autographed by Brady Hoke. I left with a first degree shoulder separation that took several weeks to heal.

I've also been trying to teach my son how to golf. At the end of one trip to the driving range, I thought I'd show off by swinging at the last ball with as much force as possible. I succeeded not only in sending my ball into orbit, but also in tearing my right tricep so badly that it hurt for a month just to pull open a door.

Of course, some injuries occur from simple overuse at the gym, and scheduled rest is indispensable for any fitness enthusiast. With kids though, there's never really any down time. I've been away from the gym for about a week now, trying to get the bursitis in my left elbow to go away. However, my son needed me to set up his basketball hoop in the driveway. The process sent shooting pain through my elbow multiple times, probably resetting my healing to day one.

So, I have advice for parents who also want to hit the gym with some regularity. First, make sure you're lifting weights light enough to complete at least 10 reps per set. Anything heavier than that just makes you too fragile and injury-prone. With no margin for error, you'll also need to stop doing gym activities that have caused you strains and sprains in the past. I love the tricep press machine, but giving my elbow time to heal is just too complicated.

Finally, set some limits: I told my daughter that when she hits 60 pounds, there's no more getting carried around on my shoulders. There was some foot stomping and hands on hips … yet another thing she can blame on her brother, I guess.

## When Truth Is Stranger than Fiction

There are a few really astounding gym incidents that I've been able only to hear about, rather than witness firsthand. For example, there are variations on the collarless barbell: A guy doing bench presses with three plates on each side pushes up unevenly; the bar tips to one side, all three plates spill off the barbell, the bar seesaws wildly through the air, and the three plates on the other side go crashing to the ground. You'll also come across the barbell catapult when someone unloads a barbell by first stripping all the plates from just one side.

(The most exciting thing to happen between me and a barbell occurred during a set of upright rows. A woman, distracted by a conversation with her boyfriend, speared herself by walking into the end of my barbell.)

I read somewhere that the reason truth is even stranger than fiction is because fiction is governed by probabilities. Now here's an incident reported on a bodybuilding site that I couldn't have even imagined:

> There was this other guy who was benching about 200 pounds. The benches were arranged along a big window that leads out to the carpark … When you lay down, the

window is behind your head. So, the guy finishes his final rep, but misses the "hooks" or whatever you call them on his bench. The bar flew crashing through the window and rolled down the carpark.

I believe it was Albert Einstein who said that the difference between stupidity and genius is that genius has its limits.

## Fearsome

Fear can be a positive force in the gym. For example, fear that an uneven lift could catapult your weight plates across the gym encourages you to secure your barbell collars. On a primal level, there's fear of rejection – even fear of death – that motivates you to go to the gym in the first place. But along the fear spectrum, you can head into a place where the feeling is less useful. If you're lifting heavy, your fear of injury increases your concentration, but might at the same time cause you to cut short your range of motion. In my case, when I perform low bar squats (Rippetoe style), my fear of the weight sometimes causes me to slide the lift forward onto my quads - where it's more comfortable, rather than back onto my weaker hamstrings and glutes - where the form is right.

At the far end of the fear spectrum resides personal trainers, and the functional training fad. As I've noted before:

> It seems like every trainer is trying to see how much "functional/balancing" crap they can use on new trainees … They jump up and down on benches, use a medicine ball and other toys.

Today, I saw a trainer order his client to perform history's most awkward set of push-ups. He instructed the poor woman to rest her shins across the top of a giant swiss ball, while she gripped two handles placed on the floor below. After mounting the wobbly ball, the terrified woman cried out: "Hold me, I'm afraid!"

Now, I question how much intensity can be directed into a set when you're training in fear. But regardless, the client completed the movement, dismounted, and then summed up in one sentence the entire state of functional fitness. "Well," she said, "it's not too bad if you hold me."

# 4 THE PEOPLE WHO INTERFERE WITH YOUR WORKOUT

## The Entire Facility Is Not Your Personal Gym Locker

A serious pet peeve of mine is some people's need to rest their workout gear - water bottles, towels, training logs - on top of nearby gym equipment rather than on the gym floor. Is this some form of unfathomable laziness (after pushing out a set of dumbbell presses, you're so depleted you can't bend over to grab your water)? Or is this an irrational hygiene issue? (The floor might be dusty, but it's not warm and sweaty.)

In either case, regarding each piece of gym equipment as an extension of your own gym locker is astonishingly self-absorbed. Stuff on a piece of equipment is, not surprisingly, the international fitness sign for "item in use." Just because no one is currently using that incline bench doesn't mean that someone very soon wouldn't like to use that bench.

This equipment-as-hat-rack issue has reached such crisis proportions that I have taken on the role of equipment vigilante. I have stopped pointing to junk on a machine I want to use and asking politely, "is this yours?" Rather, depending upon the size of relevant junk owner, I either gently remove the offending items or roughly sweep the stuff onto the floor. Almost always, people get the hint.

Today, I was ready to use the gym's ab bench. Some dude sitting in an adjacent machine had decided his gym bag was simply too special to leave next to him on the ground. He had looped the bag's strap over the ab bench's elevated footrest so that the bag dangled safely above the gym floor. I unhooked his gym bag, dropped it onto the floor, and settled into the ab bench. Looking confused, this guy scooped up his bag, walked it over to a neighboring back machine, and crammed it between two of the machine's metal posts.

I give up.

## The Broken Windows Theory of Health Clubs

All this talk of barbells sailing through actual gym windows got me thinking about sociologists' Theory of Broken Windows.

Some researchers believe that municipalities can prevent serious crime by addressing problems when they are small: Repair broken windows quickly and vandals are much less likely to break more windows or do further damage. New York City applied this theory on a wide scale in the 1990s, cracking down on turnstile jumpers, public drunkenness, urinators, and the rest. Rates of both petty and serious crime fell.

I wish that gyms would adopt a similar approach to their facilities.

I belong to two gyms with equipment of similar quality. Gym A is well lit, the machines sit atop new carpeting, and management is responsive to comments dropped in the prominently displayed Suggestion Box. As you would imagine, members cooperate when it comes to re-racking weights, sharing equipment, and attractive women aren't scared away. At Gym B, the carpet is coming apart in patches all over the place. Weight plates load down unoccupied machines. Workouts often include a five minute hunt for matching dumbbells. And of course, the membership roll provides marvelous fodder for this blog.

But here's the thing: It's really a bunch of small details that lead to a sustainable business versus a place in decline. If you don't vacuum the floor enough, if you don't promptly repair broken equipment, members receive a clear message about how to treat the club. At some point, you might even experience actual crime: equipment that can fit inside a gym bag starts to disappear (barbell collars, cable machine handles, small weight plates). Items left in gym lockers are no longer safe. Pretty soon you've got your very own fitness version of the subway line that passes through a bad neighborhood.

The sociologists are right, at least when it comes to gyms. Run the vacuum at least once a day, clean the bathrooms, empty the trash. You might save yourself a bigger headache down the road.

## Noise Pollution

I worked out in a gym last week that had on display the biggest indoor sign I'd ever seen. It was more like a billboard, in 2000 point font, hanging above the dumbbell rack: DO NOT DROP WEIGHTS.

The dropping of weights, dumbbells in particular, seems to be one of the top etiquette issues at every gym. I too am offended when people let their dumbbells crash to the ground - but only because of the damage done to the dumbbells themselves.

Heavy dumbbells that smash into the floor at an angle will bend into a c-shape, upsetting the way they balance in your hands. The weights on battered dumbbells can also come loose from the handle, and sometimes even break off. (Good luck getting your gym to fix or replace that dumbbell anytime soon.)

I think that what gyms are rallying against, however, is the bone-rattling noise of falling iron. And here's where I say: what do you expect? I'm grateful for the gyms that furnish 100+ pound dumbbells, a rare commodity in this age of express, female-targeted health clubs. But, I can also tell you that when I reach failure at the end of a set of dumbbell bench presses, I have little control over how the weights find their way to the floor. I try to ensure that the dumbbells hit flat, to avoid breaking the equipment. Beyond that, I just want to make sure that they don't tear my arms off on the way down.

I used to work out at a gym located on the second floor of a small strip mall. I was scolded several times by management for all my clanging and banging doing deadlifts with a 345 pound barbell. It wasn't the gym that cared about the noise, however, but the poor tenants on the first floor who endured the sounds of an avalanche all day long.

So here's a note to landlords: don't lease space to a gym above the ground floor. And gyms: don't lease space above the ground floor if you want your members to enjoy their regular workout.

## Mirror on the Wall

Gyms tend to make too big a deal of mirror etiquette. The list of posted rules will always include something about dropping weights, some gym-specific oddball rule like "No beverages except water allowed on the gym floor," and then something about not interfering with members' line-of-sight to the wall mirror.

I'm a big fan of watching myself in the mirror. Yes, the guy staring back at me is strikingly handsome. But as important, the feedback helps me perfect my form, and even helps with balance.

As a responsible gym user, I do my best to avoid stepping in front of others while they're in the middle of a set. If nothing else, I'm sensitive to the way this distraction can break one's concentration. Nevertheless, there are limits to mirror etiquette in a public gym, and I accept that fact on both sides of the equation.

Of course, some people are just plain jerks. A couple of days ago, I backed away from my squat rack and began a heavy set of the most painful move in the business. This guy – chatting into his Bluetooth – walked across the back of my squat rack, grabbed a weight plate from the far side of the rack, and then proceeded to stroll back across the space between the my rack and the wall.

Geez.

**Fight Club**

I get into a fight in the gym about once every 7 years.

Every time, it's with some steroid-addled gorilla. You know the type: a giant grouch, wearing a heavy sweatshirt and baggy running pants, acting as if the rest of us are invading his private gym.

Side note: If you're built like a Greek statue, why are you all covered up under thick fabric?

Now I'm not saying this guy wasn't huge. I'm just questioning the muscle to flab ratio. You get no points for flab.

So I'm resting between sets of incline dumbbell presses, and I hear someone behind me start barking out threats.

"I'm letting you know I'm coming through right now and if you don't move that bench you're going to get hurt."

"Excuse me?"

"You've got that bench way too close to the dumbbell rack and I'm not going to wait for you. It's called etiquette!"

Now technically, this butthead was right. The gym is cluttered with equipment, and I found a sliver of free space directly in front of the 70s, 75s and 80s. But what's the expression – you catch more flies with honey than with vinegar?

Besides, telling me I'm in breach of gym etiquette is like telling Martha Stewart she's put the salad fork in the wrong place. Of course, this confrontation wasn't about etiquette at all, but about my simply being in his way.

In my pump-induced fantasy, I considered taking this jerk on. Every guy in the middle of his workout imagines he's Hulk Hogan, right? I also thought it would be interesting to see two guys with lactic acid-filled shoulders struggle to lift their arms, let alone fight.

But in the end, I decided it would be best to just move. You know, literally to come back and fight another day.

Later on, I looked across the crowded gym to see what this model of health club etiquette was up to. He was working out on one of the machines, with his gym bag and water bottles spread all over a nearby bench.

**Top 10 Reasons to Switch Gyms**

The most important factor in deciding which gym to join is - let's face it - proximity. I have heard of guys that drive 20 or 30 miles to their gym of choice, something out of the question for those of us planning to keep our day jobs. Still, there are definitely occasions when it makes sense to drive just a little farther.

10. Inappropriate use of the sauna and steam facilities. Or some variation. I don't want to talk about it.

9. Three of the four 80 pound dumbbells are missing. Then one day, all the 80 pound dumbbells are missing.

8. The general manager is arrested for stealing people's identities off their membership contracts.

7. A sign reading "service required" now hangs from all three StairMasters.

6. Too many members arrive in packs of four. This is the Dreaded Foursome: loud and menacing, they take over large sections of the gym and excel at getting in the way.

5. New TVs are installed and hung from the ceiling. (What's wrong with that you ask? How about when they're hung so low that you smash them with your barbell during overhead presses.)

4. The gym decides to rearrange the equipment. This never ends well. Benches will now wobble on uneven sections of floor, lines of sight to the mirror are impaired, and somehow my favorite old-school machine always disappears. (This activity is also known as rearranging the deck chairs on the Titanic.)

3. You get busted for letting your roommate "borrow" your membership card.

2. The manager reprimands you for deadlifting too loudly.

1. Your kid urinates all over the floor of the day care center.

---

Two other opportune times to switch gyms, though I haven't experienced them personally, would be when you get tossed out of the gym for grunting too loudly (true story – reported by CBS New York), and when you accidentally launch a 200 pound barbell through the gym window.

**Sound Effects**

I consider myself something of a gym connoisseur. If you count all the college gyms, Gold's Gyms, government-owned gyms and hotel gyms I have worked out in at least once, I must have sampled at least 100 centers of fitness. And regardless of the quality of the facility, they all seem to struggle in at least one area: music.

I remember one gym where my hardcore leg workout was derailed by some shrieking rock song about ways to murder Jesus. The whole experience was so unsettling that I filed a complaint in the gym's suggestion box. The gym posted my complaint and wrote that I should have just come to the front desk and asked them to change the station. I thought this was a surprisingly fair response. But still, I don't want to have to interrupt my workout (leave the equipment, climb the stairs, find a manager) just to go futz with the radio.

The easy listening music pumped through some gyms is another workout killer. I mean, Barry Manilow's very intent is to relax you, lower your stress levels and lull you to sleep. Whatever intensity and fire you brought to fuel your workout is drained just on the walk from the check-in desk to the locker room.

Painfully loud music is as big a distraction as an afternoon of love songs. The risk of hearing damage was even the topic of a Muscle and Fitness article a few years ago.

So how about just plain off? I used to think that gyms could do the most with the least amount of noise. If you need music during your workout, bring your own headset. (Many members do in fact use their own iPods anyway – why force competing music on them?) But after experiencing the silence of gyms with broken stereos, I've changed my tune. Gym music has the wonderful effect of drowning out the frivolous conversations taking place between personal trainer and housewife, pick-up artist and target, old college roommates, or any two people discussing flab, sweat, food, fatigue, pain, cable television or the weather.

So here's my recipe: top-40 music, turned to medium volume. Like the sign of any good compromise, everyone will be slightly unhappy. But, I won't feel the need to file any more complaints.

## Taking a Hint

I get very nervous when I have to host a dinner party. My fear has nothing to do with the food prep or social anxiety, however. I am simply focused on making sure everyone leaves my house promptly when the party is over.

I have a few tools available to give people the hint. I'm a huge fan of loudly collecting everyone's plates and silverware, sometimes taking the dinnerware right out of my guests' hands. I also don't hesitate to start turning off lights. Finally, there's something I learned from my father, the best in the business when it comes to killing a party. When all else fails, I just shut off the air conditioner. You're much better off enduring a little discomfort now than entertaining long into the night.

When I'm at the gym, I feel like a guest at my own party after the dessert has been served. It's obvious they want me to leave, and for good reason:

The success of gym economics depends upon signing up members that never show. What possible good does it do to have someone like me as a member - someone who constantly pushes the equipment to its limits, consumes handfuls of paper towels to wipe off sweat, and runs up the water bill with long hot showers?

To be sure, gym managers have their own ways to give me the hint. They often blast irritating music, though I've become fairly immune to that maneuver. They also love having their cleaning crew run the vacuum right next to my bench while I'm doing sets of heavy presses. Today, they unveiled a new tactic: Between a set of squats, they sent an exterminator over to my rack to spray pesticide all along the wall.

**Emergency Bailout**

Several years ago, a friend and I were driving at night down the main strip that cuts through Charlottesville, VA. A severe electrical storm suddenly killed the power to much of the city, including the traffic lights at some busy crossroads. As we slowed near one major intersection, we were relieved to see that a policeman down the road recognized the problem, switching on his emergency lights as he approached. Dumbfounded, we watched as the police car continued to accelerate, speeding through the intersection before its lights flipped back off, leaving the rest of us to fend for ourselves.

Yesterday, a gym staff member noticed me struggling with the hip pad adjustment on the hyperextension bench. I was trying to figure out which bolts I could tighten by hand, if only to stabilize this hunk of junk for a couple of sets.

The fellow approached and said: "For your height, the pad should probably be set at number two."

"Actually," I said, "I'm concerned that the entire piece of equipment is about to fall apart."

"Well, hmm," he said, "it does look like it should probably be tightened. I guess …" He looked up as if someone had called his name. The guy began drifting off towards another part of the gym, leaving me to fend for myself as I continued with my battlefield repair.

## Warm Up

Though health clubs often spend lavishly to make the gym experience more pleasant, I'd rather see the money put towards making the time more productive. For example, I appreciate the unlimited supply of gym towels, but I'd just as soon have my sweat drip all over a new StairMaster. Likewise, I enjoy watching SportsCenter in the locker room, but I'd prefer to make my own highlights with a better leg press machine. In fact, I'd crap in a gym's outhouse and shower in recycled seawater if it meant I could establish a long term relationship with my favorite equipment.

There is one gym amenity, however, that is absolutely indispensable: the sauna.

Years ago, during my first winter in Ann Arbor, I discovered the best way to begin a pre-workout warm up: head directly from the outside into the rec center's sauna. I stripped off my ski hat, gloves and parka only after I was stationed securely inside the heated cabin. (Bonus fact: MSN Weather says average January temperatures in Ann Arbor are colder than in Anchorage, AK.)

Though the weather I'm dealing with today doesn't quite rival the Rust Belt, I frequent gyms whose approach to the sauna still leaves me cold. At one gym, an out-of-order sign has hung from the wood door since October; another gym's sauna shuts itself off after about 20 minutes and requires a manual re-start (a huge disappointment if you're the first to enter); a third gym has no sauna at all.

By its nature, a gym is a cold place, filled with iron bars, vinyl-covered equipment pads and high drafty ceilings. Furthermore, when I work out during lunch, my gym clothes have been sitting in a parked car for hours; imagine the exact opposite sensation of putting on clothes fresh out of the dryer. In total, my deepening chill isn't just uncomfortable, it's downright dangerous: cold muscles don't react well with heavy weights.

With the sauna unavailable, I've developed a new strategy for generating locker room warmth: I point the nozzle of an electric hand dryer skyward, pull my shirt over the vent, and gleefully press the button.

## Ready to Go

Whenever a holiday approaches, I'm reminded of my old swim coach's attitude toward days off. When a teammate asked in early summer whether we'd have practice on Independence Day, my coach said: "The Russians have practice on July 4th, as do the Germans … you can bet we'll be practicing too!"

Years later, it occurred to me that every athlete celebrates *an* Independence Day. During the course of a year, I'm sure that national holidays worldwide interfere with the same number of training days. Over time, workouts missed due to illness or injury probably even themselves out too. What I can't account for, however, are training disparities related to fitness center disasters.

It's never a good sign when you turn into your gym's parking lot and find two fire trucks sitting outside the club's front door. As I sense my workout slipping away, I start to descend through the five stages of grief: Denial (maybe the entire firehouse decided to exercise right now?); anger (Whiskey Tango Foxtrot! As if my workouts aren't already challenging enough!); then bargaining (I'm here only for the treadmill, so I'm fine if the free weight area has burned to the ground). Inside, I learn that an electrical circuit has blown, so the gym remains open for everything except equipment that plugs into a socket, like a treadmill.

As I slink back out of the facility with my gym bag unopened, my depression gives way to acceptance: There's got to be a vacation day somewhere in the world, right?

**Focus Group**

Due to our lack of skill, my golfing buddy and I usually play a scramble. After each stroke, we both take our next swing from the preferred location of the better ball. I remember one hole when my friend blasted his drive almost 300 yards: his ball traveled 150 yards straight and then 150 yards right, landing deep in the woods. I launched my drive straight but sky-high, causing the ball to plug hard against the wall of a sand trap. Someone in our foursome, unable to contain his schadenfreude, yelled out, "And that's your preferred drive!"

Golf is a sport that requires focus and concentration, just like serious exercise. I've long believed that proper conditioning is not just a measure of fitness, but also an ability to block out a gym's countless distractions. Frankly, I don't see how you can achieve one without the other. Just take a look at a typical week of assaults on my senses.

**Sight**: On Monday, I pushed open the door of my gym and walked into a cave. The fellow at the front desk asked my forgiveness for the power outage, and invited me to work out anyway. Dude: no apology necessary - I'm just delighted the front door is unlocked. The rest is up to me.

**Sound**: How about working out while a fire alarm shrieks endlessly? (Same gym, same time.)

**Smell**: On Wednesday, my jump rope and I were met at the threshold of the aerobics room by the health club version of tear gas: a repairman was applying industrial lubricant to a dozen stationary bikes. I counted on my clean-running liver to process the toxic fumes at the same rate I inhaled them.

**Touch**: On Friday, the gym I used has its free weight area built on some kind of plywood platform. When I perform heavy squats, I can feel the floor sag under the weight of each rep.

Now I know what you're thinking: The distractions at the beginning of the week were just a coincidence, but an unstable floor is a permanent feature. Shouldn't a weak base be motivation enough to go find a new club?

Actually, this facility is my preferred gym.

## No Class

I admit there's one part of the gym experience with which I have no experience: aerobics classes. I've always figured that my own training is far more intense than whatever workout the instructor regresses to the mean. I'd also rather control my own pace and intervals of rest. Regardless, I do spend a great deal of time in the aerobics room – the mirrors and wood floor create the perfect environment for jumping rope. And whenever I jump rope prior to the start of an aerobics class, I am a witness to some incredibly bizarre behavior.

First of all, many members turn their aerobics class into a major half-day activity. People start showing up nearly two hours early to reserve their favorite spots on the floor, marking their territory with the full aerobics complement of step, weights and mat. The scene begins to resemble the unwashed crowd waiting outside early on Black Friday morning. One woman sits atop her step with a book; another naps along her mat. I'm sure that soon someone will whip out a portable stove top and begin cooking breakfast.

I can only assume that the line of sight to the instructor or to the mirror is the cornerstone of the entire enterprise. I have watched one woman on several occasions move her aerobics gear as close to the front of the room as possible – where I happened to be swinging a thin plastic tube at multiple revolutions per second. Even as my rope is smacking against her step, she continues in oblivion to load the rest of her gear into position. When she comes back for her class an hour later, her equipment is mysteriously touching the back wall.

This morning, I watched the level of aerobics egocentrism reach a new high. A guy setting up his station decided that the aerobics room dumbbells weren't heavy enough for him. So he went out to the regular gym dumbbell rack, helped himself to the pair of 20s and 25s, and walked them back to his station. These community dumbbells, useful for bicep curls, forearm work and shoulder laterals, began collecting dust on the floor of the aerobics room - an hour before the class even started.

## In Decline

The decline bench should be a place to do great work. Tricep extensions performed on a decline bench force your arms to move under constant tension; Russian twists on a decline build rotational strength and grow obliques that look like armor; decline dumbbell presses cover a huge range of motion and focus the load almost exclusively on your pecs. (I've read that decline dumbbell presses might be the perfect chest exercise.)

Unfortunately, gyms and equipment manufacturers have conspired to turn the decline bench into just more weight room clutter.

Almost every decline bench I've ever climbed onto makes me seasick. I don't know whether to blame the gyms that won't tighten the pivotal bolt, or manufacturers that throw together such an unstable piece of equipment. Regardless, every chest day, I find myself rolling back and forth as I work to press up two heavy dumbbells.

Today, I mounted a decline bench that actually got the stability right. It was designed, however, without any consideration for the proportions of the human body. The leg pads were fixed at least 12 inches too high, so that my butt and low back were pulled off the bench. The whole position was so insecure that as soon as I started pressing, I slid right down the slope of the decline.

I did find a gym once with a good decline bench. Two in fact, side by side.

They were solid, stable, ready to go. Of course, they were located up a long flight of stairs and down the hall, impossibly far from the gym's dumbbell rack.

## Out of Order

There has been a flurry of gym openings in my city recently, a development I approach with a mix of optimism and trepidation. An established gym, by its very existence, discourages competitors from opening nearby; a gym in operation also (tries to) dominate the membership market in a three to five mile radius. Bottom line: If a couple local gyms clutter up their floors with second-rate equipment and stylish contraptions, I am pretty much condemned to years of unsatisfying workouts.

My only other option, currently in practice, is to drive all over the area with a keychain full of gyms' plastic barcodes. When individual gyms fail to offer an adequate equipment selection, I have to join multiple gyms (or a club with multiple locations) and string together a powerhouse program one machine at a time.

For the record, here are four core pieces of equipment every serious health club should offer (also a good checklist when scouting a new facility):

- Free standing dip bars, thick enough to remain stiff under the load of weighted dips
- Seated pulley row machine
- A stable decline bench
- A quality leg press machine

I know this list seems simple enough, close to the assortment you'd find in the basements or garages of many homes. However, between the dozen gyms to which I've belonged, and the scores more in which I've worked out, I know of exactly one gym, in Fairfax, Co. Virginia, that has implemented this list 4-for-4. Of course, when that gym underwent a renovation a few years ago, they got rid of the dip bars and the leg press – and me.

Although I travel to multiple gyms weekly, I've never considered driving to separate gyms for the same workout. I couldn't imagine starting to exercise in one location, and finding something so deficient that I'd have to finish somewhere else. Well, here we go. Let's just say that today, I had a lot of bran cereal for breakfast; in the middle of my workout, I found in the men's locker room this sign taped to the door of both bathroom stalls:

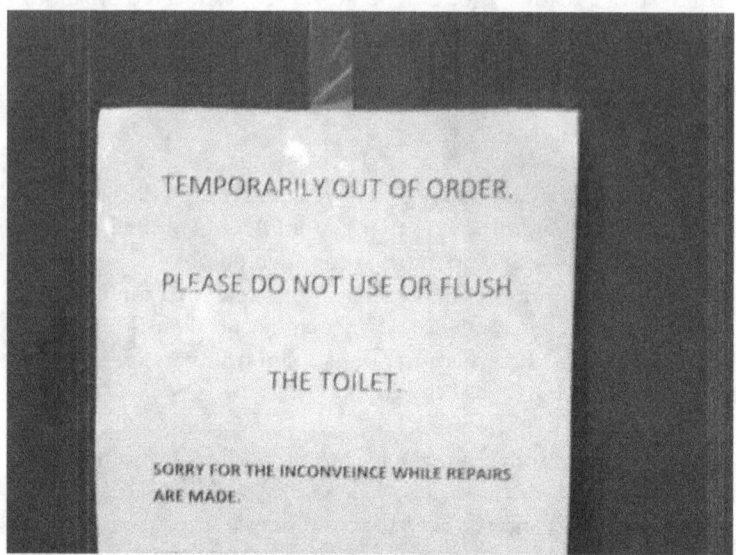

## Bump and Run

For the past few years I've participated in an annual 5K run sponsored by a nearby town. Since the course is the same each year, I use the race as an annual benchmark of my level of fitness. I've also experimented with listening to music during the race, taking into account issues of etiquette, safety, and whether it's even desirable to tune out the event. I can report that whatever the drawbacks, earphones will indeed help you go much faster.

The race organizers do a nice job at the starting line trying to separate the faster runners from the slower folks. Several large signs clearly indicate where you're supposed to stand based on your typical pace per mile. Each group goes off in a staggered start separated by a minute or so.

Although this athletic honor system should help streamline the race, the whole arrangement breaks down under actual event conditions. Pumped full of pre-race adrenaline, people who have never run three miles in less than 30 minutes conclude they're going to streak down the course at an eight minute pace. Likewise, you have folks with no conditioning at all that decide to accompany their more fitness-oriented spouse or relative at the starting line.

Everything would be fine if these people, totally gassed by 1,000 meters, drifted off towards the sidewalk in a courteous and controlled fashion.

Unfortunately for the rest of us, they crash suddenly and stop right in your path. For those of us in the third or fourth wave of runners, the first half of the race is most notable for its frequent collisions and for weaving around the widespread traffic jams. In fact, the beginning of the race encapsulates everything wrong with the state of fitness today: People with unrealistic expectations starting too fast, burning themselves out, all while getting in the way of folks trying to train seriously.

There's also fun to be had at the water stations at miles one and two of the course. Now, I imagine the race organizers set up these stations only for liability purposes or because it's required by some county code. As a practical matter, do you really need to suck down a pint of water nine minutes into your jog? I'm serious – are people normally crazy with thirst after four laps around a track? I know that I haven't even started to sweat yet at this point in my workout. Regardless, runners swarm the tables and fling their empty cups all over the road. In particular, I like watching the guys who grab a cup of water in each hand and pour it over their heads, like they're heading into the final stage of a triathlon.

## The Key Thing

It turns out that one of the biggest obstacles to having a good workout is just getting through the gym's front door. Now I don't mean this in a motivational or philosophical sense – I mean literally having a gym employee remember to get out of bed in the morning and go unlock the front door.

Over the course of my fitness career, I've seen dozens of gym parking lots fill up with restless and angry members, regardless of the city or the brand. In fact, I belong to more than one gym, in part so I can escape fiascos like the one I came across today.

Given all the ways gyms try to entice people to join, I think I'd start my own franchise with an access guarantee and the most basic of slogans: "We open on time." (I should also mention my idea for a gym in Washington D.C. near the U.S. Capitol called, "The House of Reps.")

In any event, whenever my workout gets sidetracked by a gym's deadbolt, I often consider trashing them on the Internet, either lighting them up on Twitter or naming names on this blog. But in reality, I don't think damaging their business helps me in the long run. In point of fact, I need all my gyms to stay open, so that one of them does indeed remain open.

# 5 THE PEOLE WHO DISTRACT YOU FROM YOUR WORKOUT

## Getting In On the Action

One of the most frustrating aspects of staying fit is having my workout impaired not by my own lethargy, but by problems with equipment in the gym. I've often wondered about a gym's process for selecting its equipment. Does anyone with fitness experience actually try out the equipment first, or are they buying based just on price, or the slickness of a website? And even more fundamentally, what goes on exactly at the companies that manufacture gym equipment? Do the engineers and designers have any personal history pushing, pulling and squeezing in the gym? Does anyone actually sit in the prototype and blast out a few reps before it gets mass produced and shipped out the door?

A machine's "action" – the way the resistance rises and falls with the movement – should, I think, simulate the feel of an oar pulling through the water: smooth, constant, uniform. What you often get, however, are machines that force you to fight against the resistance as much as the weights themselves. Almost every gym comes equipped with a Smith machine that sticks and snags all the way down and all the way up; a fly machine with tension that appears and disappears throughout the range of motion; and a plain wacky cable machine that must have a gremlin inside playing with the weight stack. This issue extends to even some of the cheaper treadmills that have the feel of running under water.

Equally frustrating, but more dangerous, is the lack of stability plaguing so much equipment. Too often I can grab the top of an incline bench's pad and rock it side to side with just my hand; what do you think might happen when I'm lying on the same bench pushing hard against two monster dumbbells? I've actually dropped a dime in between a preacher bench's support beam and shaft to secure the arm pad in place. And I can't tell you how many shims I've made from folded up paper towels in a desperate attempt to steady the legs on some bench or machine.

Note to gyms: ever notice how the feet on the base of every machine has holes in it? That's so you can take a drill and a screw and secure the equipment to the floor. I have worked out in gyms that care enough to bolt down their equipment, and let me tell you: it's incredible. There is no better feeling in the gym than pushing up against some massive weight with exclusive focus on completing the rep.

Now back to the factory. What is so complicated about the padding for your basic flat bench? I've been forced to bench press on pads so cushy they should be sold as mattresses. I've done presses on pads so wide they stop my arms from reaching a full stretch at the bottom of my lift. And this: Why did you guys make a calf raise machine that forces my feet so far forward of the shoulder pads that I have no leverage to perform the lift at all? Why did you build the barbell supports on your preacher curl bench in a place that blocks a full extension of my arms? And … really … why are your dumbbells so easily bent out of shape when dropped hard against the floor? I used a gym once where each dumbbell seemed to be forged as one solid piece of iron - that's how you make your dumbbells indestructible.

In fairness, there is a huge expense associated with quality gym equipment. Between the cost of raw metal and the chunk set aside for the lawyers, it's amazing the economics of fitness work at all. Nevertheless, I declare myself available to any gym equipment manufacturer as an official machine tester. Who knows, if the stuff actually works, folks might be more inclined to buy it.

## Halloween in January

You can tell a lot about a person's commitment to fitness by how he or she dresses in the gym. In this case, more really is less. The more colorful, stylish and expensive the getup, the less likely you will see that person at the gym next month, or even next week.

But what to make of the guy who comes to workout dressed like he's teeing off at Augusta National? I'm talking about the collared shirt, leather belt, slacks and shoes that sparkle under the gym lighting. This is not the fellow dressed in his business casual because he forgot to pack his gym clothes. I'm referring to the guy who looks into his closet on a Sunday morning and thinks that workout gear ought to be dry cleaned.

On the female side, I'm both appreciative of and confounded by the attire that looks like it was lifted from a Picasso painting. These one piece outfits stretch over the whole body, with geometric chunks missing from the back, stomach and side of the leg. What really perplexes me, however, are the women (often the same) who come to the gym in full prom makeup. I decided to consult an expert.

Me: Honey, what is the deal with the women wearing a ton of makeup at the gym? (Again, I'm referring to a Sunday morning, not coming from work.)

Honey: Yeah, I know what you mean.

Me: But wouldn't all the makeup run down your face once you start sweating?

Honey: What makes you think they break a sweat?

Right. Now I get it.

**International Health Emergency**

During my research for this book, I came across a thread at the Men's Health's U.K. discussion board about ridiculous behavior at the gym. Sounds like stupidity at the club is something of a global epidemic. A few highlights.

Cell phone abuse:

> Right fellas, I've been working out for 4/5 years now and I have seen a lot of funny/stupid stuff in the gym, but today's incident takes the biscuit. I was coming out of the changing rooms and I saw a guy on his mobile phone ... normal enough so far you might say. Well how about the fact that he was also on a rowing machine and rowing one handed???

> ... One day when one of these idiots was on the running machine and as usual on his mobile phone, he was getting

rather animated and dropped his phone. Human instinct being what it is he quickly reached down to try and catch it as he did he forgot to keep moving his legs, anyway there is one almighty crash as his face hits the treadmill and he gets flung off the back and is laying in a heap at the end ... bloodied nose and serious bruised ego, but he only tried to style it out, went back on the runner for about 30 sec's, hobbling, then gave up, I laughed so hard I nearly pissed myself.

Treadmill issues:

I was on a treadmill once and the guy next to me thought he'd jam his speed up to the max ... next thing I know he's making some god almighty noises and trying desperately to stab at the controls while continuing to run. Several seconds later just when I thought this guy's head was gonna blow off he managed to slam his hand down on the emergency stop and the sudden deceleration launched him into the mirror in front of the machine ... don't you just hate trying to cover up a major attack of hysterics?!?!

On bad form:

This one male was doing dumbbell lateral raises (shoulders) with weights far too heavy. In order to raise the left one he leant to the right then, breathed in, took two massive steps left, screamed, swung them above his head, and brought them down in front of him, in an almost windmill action ... my god.

General absurdity:

My old gym had not long opened when I joined and they insist on showing people around. There was a salesman who wanted to show off the swimming pool which you had to access through the changing room. While he was showing a group of attractive young women around he made the mistake of not telling them he would meet them around the other side of the changing rooms. So 6 teenage students followed, walking boldly through the men's changing room while around 20 of us had just finished a circuit training session.

## My Confession

I have a confession. My story about the craziest thing I'd seen in the gym wasn't entirely truthful. Don't get me wrong: the contents of the post were completely factual – there is no need to embellish anything. Nevertheless, I have seen one spectacle far more preposterous than anything I've discussed previously. I simply didn't have the confidence to share it until now.

What I saw filled me with such stupefaction that I can preface it only by quoting H. L. Mencken: "It is so bad that a sort of grandeur creeps into it."

When this guy rolled a fully inflated exercise ball beside a couple heavy dumbbells, I thought his next movement must have been prescribed by a doctor or physical therapist. Why else would any sane person kneel on top of an exercise ball, fight for balance, then bring two huge dumbbells up to shoulder height and begin pressing? Perhaps there was something happening that I simply didn't understand.

I found this exercise ludicrous from just the perspective of safety. The overloaded ball could burst. It could suddenly roll, sending a man attached to two large dumbbells flying in any direction. Even a small shift would instantly rip up his rotator cuff.

I planned on keeping all this secret until I had an edifying email exchange with a fellow gym-traveler. He reported:

> Next to a group of people doing various mat exercises a guy plunks down the biggest swiss ball available, fetches two 15kg dumbbells and proceeds to *stand* on the swiss ball. He balanced himself for about 10 minutes before raising the dumbbells above his head. Needless to say not long after he got on the swiss ball a massive space around him formed. It was like the parting of the sea!

The good news is I now realize that exercise ball abuse is part of the gymsanity experience. The bad news is that gym guests are even bigger idiots than I thought.

## The Rest of the Story

My nightmare featuring crazed gym ball users keeps getting worse. They guy standing on the exercise ball with his dumbbells? I guess balance really is an issue:

So I saw the guy on the swiss ball again today doing bicep curls, but this time he fell off, twice ... The first time, I heard a loud clang as the guy managed to catch himself before falling right onto me by grabbing the top of the rack. The second time thankfully no one was near him as he had to actually jump off the ball and land awkwardly to the side of the ball. Scary stuff!

When this guy ends up seriously hurting himself, the key question becomes: Will he sue the swiss ball manufacturer because of the product's round, unstable shape?

I ask because my gym printed out an article on just this topic and taped it to the mirror nearest its collection of exercise balls. An excerpt:

> A man claims that an exercise ball he was using in a fitness program at a Jacksonville YMCA exploded while he was on it, sending him to a hospital with serious injuries and changing his life. The man said he broke both wrists and one forearm and injured both shoulders when the ball blew up like a balloon as he was on it while using about 150 pounds of weights ... Nearly two years later, he and his wife are filing a lawsuit against both the manufacturer of the ball and the YMCA.

My gym added a handwritten note at the bottom of the article: *Use at your own risk.*

## Top 10 Things Not To Do At a Gym Water Fountain

My sister thinks that the commotion surrounding a gym water fountain is just knee-slapping hilarious, and that this blog would be incomplete without a more thorough analysis. Ok, Elana, here you go:

10. Take a big gulp of water, turn around, and cough into the face of the person waiting behind you.

9. Empty the remnants of your sports drink into the fountain, especially if it's red (tends to streak like the blood from snot or spit; see 8-7). Come to think of it, I don't want to see pools of orange or green either.

8. Spit in the fountain.

7. Blow your nose in the fountain.

6. Bathe in the water fountain. This means no coming out of the spinning room and rinsing your whole face in the fountain stream.

5. Hog the water fountain. If you need to fill up your water bottle, be considerate of the people waiting for a quick sip behind you.

4. Hold a conversation right in front of the water fountain.

3. Never, ever change the stupid newspaper article hung directly behind the water fountain.

2. Rinse out your Tupperware, yogurt container or any other item holding food residue in the fountain.

1.  Fail to report/fix water as hot as piss coming out of the fountain.

---

A couple readers have suggested an 11th thing not to do at a gym water fountain: put your mouth over the entire spout like you're trying to suck the water straight out of the pipe. I guess this is akin to double-dipping your chip; it's like putting your entire mouth in the bowl. In any event, it's gross.

Thanks for sharing.

**Customer Service**

Today at the gym I watched a personal trainer and his beginner client spend a good 10 minutes exploring the all-important torso twist machine. Don't get me wrong - I'm all for a well-defined set of internal obliques. But I have to believe there are better places in the gym for this novice to spend his time, and money.

Personal trainers are expensive. Just one session can cost double or triple the price of an entire month's gym membership. Are people getting their money's worth?  Not according to one comment I read on a bodybuilding site.

> Some of the training stuff that goes on at my gym these
> days drives me nuts. It seems like every trainer is trying to

see how much "functional/balancing" crap they can use on
new trainees … They jump up and down on benches, use
a medicine ball and other toys. If you are a seasoned
and/or experienced athlete and want to do wall squats
with a swiss ball, or incorporate the new koosh ball feet
thingies into your workout ... no problem. But shouldn't
someone that looks like they need a major overhaul start
with real weight training and some real cardio?

The dubious certification process for personal trainers accounts for some
of these misplaced priorities. I did a little research and found that over 300
different certifications exist, with many - perhaps most - earned simply by
mailing in a check.

Still, I'm beginning to think that clients are in fact quite happy to pay for
the illusion of fitness. I'm reminded of the very average couple down the
street that likes to brag about their retention of a financial planner. Perhaps
the value for gym members comes not from actual physical improvement,
but from the opportunity to start sentences with the words "my trainer."

For sure, it's the exceptional client that looks forward to a challenging
workout. True story: On my last day as a personal trainer, a client who had
been making steady gains told me he wanted my replacement to be "less of
a drill sergeant." I've also noticed that some of the loudest, most animated
conversations at my gym take place between trainer and client.
Furthermore, why does every client seem to progress through her workout
with a giant grin on her face?

I've reached the conclusion that the sorry state of personal training actually
reflects a high level of customer service. They're just giving the customer
what she wants.

## Team Effort

I've often wondered whether asking a stranger for a spot is a violation of
gym etiquette. I know that when I'm asked for a spot, I'm irritated by the
disruption in the pace of my workout and the break in concentration. I also
resent channeling my precious energy into someone else's workout, and,
considering the absurd amount of weight usually involved, putting my low
back at risk.

I'm no hypocrite: I also gave up asking for spots years ago, though mostly
because people don't understand the concept of spotting for safety.

Typically, you're just encouraging the shared lift you often see at the gym. You've got the spotter who assists his partner on the leg press by repeatedly throwing himself into the machine's carriage. Or, how about the guys performing barbell bicep curls when it's not clear who's doing the lifting and who's doing the spotting. The bottom line is that a spotter has no business touching anything unless the lifter is just plain stuck. Besides, if you're using an appropriate amount of weight, a spotter really shouldn't be necessary.

I do know that when someone else imposes a spot on you, he's definitely crossed the line of gym etiquette.

True story: I'm minding my own business, lying back on a flat bench with two heavy dumbbells. As I start my set, some guy runs up behind me, cups his hands under my elbows, and proceeds to push up on my arms through 8 or 9 reps.

A couple questions present themselves:

1) Am I supposed to thank this idiot for his counterproductive spot?

2) Why do certain people believe that proper lifting requires some kind of group hug?

**Phoning It In**

When I join a gym, I feel like it's my first day at a new job. I've got to figure out the lay of the land, such as the location of the bathroom. As important, I've got to pick up quickly on the culture. For example, at some gyms, loud grunting will earn you a dirty look from gym staff. At others, making a scene while you lift is encouraged – even admired. Regardless, at all gyms, there's one rule you have to respect: You must cooperate when someone asks you for a spot.

I've covered my objections to spotting – it interrupts the pacing of my workout; it offends my sensibilities to see someone using more weight than he can handle; on the bench press, it puts my low back in a terrible position. But most of all, if the guy benching 315+ suffers a total failure, I literally can't help. There's no way I can pull an anvil off some guy's chest.

So during my workout today, the guy next to me throws three plates onto each side of his barbell. He looks my way and says, "Hey, can you help me out." I started trudging over to my position behind his bench, but I noticed his strange expression. "Here," he says, as he hands me his phone.

"My buddy doesn't believe I can bench this weight. I need you to video this lift for me."

Finally, a spot where I can actually help.

## Follow the Money

I imagine the neat thing about being rich – and I'm talking really rich – is that you can indulge your interests in the extreme. John Travolta pursued his love of flight by earning a commercial pilot's license, then building a house attached to an airplane hangar connected to a private runway. Steve Wynn's personal art gallery includes a Picasso worth over $100 million. Likewise, Paris Hilton has a collection of over 1,000 pairs of shoes.

When my career as a swim model reaches its apogee, I'll be psyched to start furnishing my own personal gym.

Funny thing is (funny weird, not funny ha-ha) I'm having to buy things for my current club as if it were my personal gym. Not because I want to, of course, but because most gyms fail to provide even the most elementary tools of a safe and productive workout. Here's a look at some items in my gym bag:

**WD-40**: Yes, the industrial lubricant. I carry the smaller spray bottle, and have no problem whipping it out and performing my own gym maintenance. Rusty machines are a workout killer.

**Collars**: Gyms ought to provide buckets of barbell collars on the gym floor. You'd think just from a liability perspective, gyms would be eager to prevent heavy iron plates from slipping off barbells and flying through the air. I've been to gyms that make you check out collars from the front desk, or simply have none available. In any event, I'll be securing my weight plates and protecting myself from joint or tearing injuries.

**Soap**: Barbells and dumbbells accumulate germs as fast as the filthiest subway pole. If gyms aren't refilling the soap dispenser in the bathroom fast enough, at least I'm prepared.

## The Power of Positive Thinking

Recognizing that positive energy attracts more good things into your life, I'd like to share the Top 5 Most Outstanding Things I've Ever Seen at the Gym:

5) The guys who showed me how to use lifting straps properly. With the first loop, the strap goes under the bar, not your palm. Otherwise, the barbell will just slip out of your hands.

4) The guy who at about 5'9", 170 pounds, performed 7 clean, strong reps of bench presses with 115 pound dumbbells. Oh wait, that was me.

3) Saturday aerobics class, third row, purple crop top.

2) Most creative abdominal move ever: guy straps belt to waist, hooks belt into low cable pulley. He puts Frisbee-like plates under each foot, assumes a pull-up position, and brings knees to chest. Looks hard.

1) Basketball great Patrick Ewing walking on a treadmill. He's taller than the machine is long.

## A Farewell to Arms

Though technically not one of the most outstanding things I've ever seen in the gym, Arnold Schwarzenegger's visit to my high school in 1991 definitely ranks up there as one of my top moments in bodybuilding.

Arnold's limo arrived at the football field and drove the long way around the track. Finally, Arnold got out of the car. He surveyed the crowd and announced into the mike: "I see a flabalanche!"

After Arnold completed his address, the president of the senior class presented him with a school t-shirt. Arnold held up the shirt by each sleeve and declared, "I never accept a shirt without trying it on first." At this point, I thought we were about to be treated to an impromptu posing routine by the greatest bodybuilder of all time. Unfortunately, Arnold just pulled the t-shirt over what he was wearing. I guess Arnold figured that at age 43, there was no need for reality to eclipse the legend.

Still, he did not disappoint. Arnold electrified the crowd by hitting a huge double bicep pose - the most impressive thing I've ever seen in a short sleeved shirt.

Of course, Arnold's signature muscle is his bicep. He credits his arms, the peak of his biceps, with winning him championships. Nevertheless, Arnold also worked hard to build a well-balanced physique. No bodybuilder advances in the sport without symmetry among all muscle groups.

In fact, I don't think the typical fitness amateur accomplishes much without giving appropriate attention to each body part. Your respect for a fellow gym member declines real fast as your eyes shift from his bulging arms to his A-cup chest. Similarly, guys with big upper bodies betray their lack of seriousness with their scrawny bottom halves.

The general population's obsession with arms certainly makes for some pointless workouts. I'm always amazed when I can finish an entire leg routine while a couple guys take turns doing barbell bicep curls at a neighboring squat rack. Ok guys, you're right: It's the *eighth* set of curls that's going to make the difference.

## Tough Read

I'm always worried by the guys who bring bodybuilding "how-to" books onto the gym floor. My first reaction is similar to when I spot a car with a Student Driver sign: I slowly back away and give him a wide berth. Recently, I've been thinking about that scene from Spies Like Us, when Chevy Chase and Dan Aykroyd attempt an appendectomy by reading through the medical textbook they're hiding under the operating table.

I'm fairly certain that reading material has no place near exercise equipment. You know what I think of the people who do cardio while reading People. Well today, I saw a guy working out on this "cross trainer" machine (envision a seated StairMaster) with a full blown hardcover novel, complete with tassel dangling from the bookmark. The guy supported himself with his right arm, while cradling the book in his left arm. He cupped his left hand around the top of the book to keep the pages spread open.
I walked by a couple times to see if I could nonchalantly pick up the title of the novel. Unfortunately, this gentleman was bored by his workout and his book, and succeeded in brushing me off with an evil eye.

So, does this man's absent-minded, indifferent approach to his weekend hobby offend me as a bodybuilder? Actually, no. It offends me as a writer.

## Washed Away

Every morning, my gym rubs my nose in it. On my way to the locker room, the gym's layout forces me to walk past the swimming pool - a reminder not only of wasted gym fees, but also of my deeper philosophical objections to the whole activity.

Let me be blunt: Stripping down to your banana hammock and diving into the pool is probably the worst possible use of your exercise time. I say this not as some cannonball specialist, but as a former competitive swimmer, with a record at a club in Northern Virginia that still stands after 22 years.

There are the obvious drawbacks to swimming laps: the feeling of someone's snot sliding down your leg, sections of pool that seem suspiciously warm, the sight of dirty Band-Aids floating past.

There's also the problem with H2O itself. Water's cooling effect causes the body to retain, or even increase, fat stores. In water, people can twist their joints in unnatural ways, triggering all kinds of knee and shoulder injuries. And in contrast to every other form of physical activity, a pool's minimal gravity does nothing to improve bone density.

Most importantly, it's just intolerable the way chlorine damages your hair.

Regardless, if you're going to go through the hassle of submerging yourself in cold water and the annoyance of a public bath, at least try. On my way to the locker room today, I saw a guy holding a kickboard in his outstretched arms, pretending to exercise by casually walking up and down the lane.

## Mind Games

People underestimate the mental soreness that follows from serious training. Just as the anticipation of pain is as bad as pain itself, the mental preparation required for a big lift – or an entire leg day for that matter – is as exhausting as the physical workout.

I know what happens to me when mental fatigue sets in and I start to lose my concentration. I'll find myself doing presses with an 85 pound dumbbell in my right hand and an 80 pound dumbbell in my left. Or I'll absent-mindedly load my barbell with a weight unrelated to what I normally use.

Of course, loss of focus is all relative. I had the opportunity this week to watch a fellow member do his best impression of staggering home drunk.

What started as a normal walk from one machine to another ended with a sudden stumble, a flailing of limbs, and a water bottle spilling all over the floor.

At this point, you could see the wheels of indecision turning in this guy's head. Should he compound his embarrassment by grabbing some paper towels and starting to wipe from his knees? Or should he just keep moving and put as much distance as possible between himself and the incident?

I thought to myself that there was actually a third way, an old trick that I learned in the huge, anonymous lecture halls at law school. When the professor picks your name off the roll to answer some obscure question - or you happen to spill your drink all over the gym floor – just turn sideways and stare intensely at the person next to you.

**Fitness Revolution**

Although I've clearly taken sides in the ongoing conflict of gym vs. member, the strategies on both sides deserve recognition.

Gyms have the home field advantage, of course, forcing members to devise engineering marvels just to get in a decent workout. At one gym, I came across an ingenious solution to the inexcusable lack of a pull-up station.

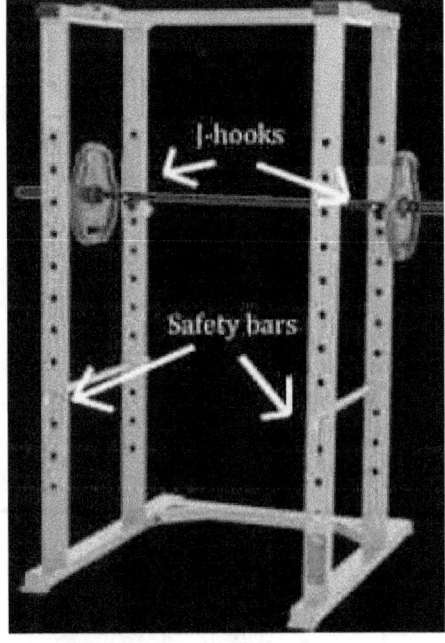

Some members had laid a barbell across the top of a squat cage and used lifting straps to fasten the bar to the frame. At a different gym, I watched a guy approach the squat rack at the beginning of his leg routine, only to find that the j-hooks had mysteriously disappeared. He moved the safety bars to shoulder height and flipped them upside-down, creating makeshift arms on the outside of the cage to prevent the bar from rolling off.

Members aren't just suffering these humiliations sitting down, however. In the sauna, I was recently stunned as one

47

gentleman got up from the bench and poured his half-finished water bottle all over the top of the electric heating unit. I don't know if he confused the geothermal rocks in an authentic Swedish sauna with the expensive box plugged into this sauna. Regardless, while everyone else looked on approvingly, I got the hell out of there.

Although members do score the occasional victory, gyms continue to innovate around crushing the spirit of their clientele. This morning, I stopped at my gym's entrance to take in a new poster touting improvements coming soon. My muscles tingled at the thought of a better leg press, a replacement for that clunker of a calf-machine, and new treadmills that don't malfunction mid-run. But then I read the details of the planned upgrades: More kettlebells, a coat of paint for the cardio room, and a renovation of the smoothie bar. Well played, indeed.

## Inquiring Minds

I don't mind when people approach me with questions between sets. Give people credit for recognizing excellence and caring enough to learn more. Lately, I've been drawing a lot of attention with my Manta Ray squat pad, and folks wanting to know if it makes squats easier. Yes it does, since the device neutralizes problems caused by the typical bent and rusty barbell. However, with the bar placed higher on your traps, you'll work harder as you're forced into better, upright form.

When it comes to strange questions, I'd have to give the gold medal to a personal trainer who once sought me out. With her client in tow, this trainer inquired about what exercise I had been doing. It was that newfangled motion called deadlifts.

Irrespective of the query, I draw the line when someone wants to chat mid-exercise. Today, I was grinding away on the StairMaster, with my headphones drowning out the pain and my sweat streaming down the handrails. Desperate for my attention, a woman began knocking hard on the base of my machine. Obviously the gym must be on fire. I couldn't really hear what this woman was saying, but the upshot was that she wanted to commend me on my workout intensity. Ironic that she didn't see herself as an impediment towards that goal.

I intended to discount this last intrusion as just another example of poor gym etiquette, but then I had an epiphany. If I had witnessed something in the gym as unusual as a person training hard, wouldn't I also seek out the nearest member to gush about it?

---

As a footnote, I'd add that violations of gym etiquette aren't limited to the gym. I was in the middle of a jog once when a car rolled up next to me and began matching my brisk 8-minute mile pace. The driver lowered her window and shouted out a question about directions.

## What's It Worth?

I've been travelling for business this week, and had to do some soul searching regarding one of life's fundamental questions: How much should I pay for a workout?

At home, my gym membership costs about $40 per month. If I go two of every three days, I'm paying an actual $2 per workout. Not bad.

Some of the more expensive gyms in my area cost up to $800 a year. Throw in an initiation fee, and with a 66 percent attendance rate, you're looking at close to $5 a workout. Kind of bad.

To me, $5 is dangerously close to real money. For five bucks, you can swill a grande latte, view a matinee, or pay for a couple gallons of gas. The discouraging part about gyms in this price range is that you're probably funding a bunch of things you never even use, like swimming pools and squash courts. You'd be much better served if the gym simply added a donkey calf raise machine to the main floor.

The maximum one-time guest fee for gyms used to hover around $10. In my heart, I figured I would pay $10 for the perfect workout: an empty gym with the latest equipment, a mix of my favorite songs playing over the speakers. Lately, however, I've seen guest fees of $15, and today, I found a gym that charged $20.

If I had to pay $20 per workout at my home gym, I'd be paying $400 per month, or almost $5,000 per year. No wonder $20 feels ridiculous.

Nevertheless, people do pay four- or even five figures for their gym memberships. Some of these clubs are built for celebrities and don't really apply. But what about the super high end place that offers cutting edge equipment, caps its membership (or number of people allowed on the floor at one time), and lets you grunt away in a spa-like environment? I have to believe that working out in a veritable penthouse would boost my motivation and reduce the agony.

Well, maybe.

## Up Scale

I don't want to talk about the circumstances, but I found myself recently in a super high end place that features a spa-like environment. You know the kind of place - where the actual gym serves as a loss leader for the club café. Is this really a better way to work out? You be the judge based on the top 10 most remarkable things I saw:

10. A dealer's Mercedes parked on front lawn with a sign on the windshield promising special offers for members.

9. A membership requirement that includes an initiation fee, an administration fee and a triple digit monthly fee.

8. An empty Perrier bottle left on the gym floor.

7. Eco-friendly showers that try to create the sensation of a regular shower by spraying a combination of 50 percent air and 50 percent water. (It just takes you twice as long to get clean.)

6. An indoor waterfall.

5. A man near the aerobics rooms balancing on his head.

4. A locker room that includes a Miami sauna and a Phoenix sauna (door on the left takes you into a wet steam, door on right is a traditional dry heat).

3. Plush leather couches stationed outside the hair salon.

2. Mobbed machines.

1. Empty squat racks.

## Coming Soon

Many years ago, before cable television, I remember seeing an amazing contraption at the house of a family friend. The dad had connected his television to his exercise bike so that the bike powered the TV. He could watch television only while converting calories into literal energy. The timing of his workouts determined what was available to him for entertainment.

Recently, my gym installed a "cardio theater," a room with a large screen facing an array of treadmills and stationary bikes. Gym members often stop at the front desk to ask "what time does the movie start?" and schedule their workouts accordingly. Today, the timing of the entertainment determines when people are available to work out.

This week's sign of the fitness apocalypse isn't just the waste of gym resources (money and floor space) now required to persuade people to break a sweat. To my mind, watching a movie while you exercise is similar to trying to read a book. If you're concentrating enough to truly follow the plot, you're not focusing adequately on the task at hand.

But regardless of the philosophical issues, I got to thinking about what films might provide the necessary workout inspiration. How about Sylvester Stallone in Rocky IV? A loop of Schwarzenegger flicks? Anything starring Sophia Vergara?

I poked my head into the theater today and saw a staff member working on the electronics. I asked her what type of movies they had loaded into the video player. "UFOs and stuff," she said.

"What do you mean?" I asked.

"Oh, end of the world movies, that kind of thing."

"Gotcha," I said. Now I'm inspired.

# 6 A LIGHTER APPROACH

## Gatekeeper

I've invested a great deal of time and thought over the years into sneaking visiting relatives into gyms. Restrictive guest policies combined with the crazy cost of one-time gym passes means there's real pressure to try and outthink the front desk staff.

My uncle is a master in this area. He's one of those guys who needs only some kind of identification – I've seen him use a library card – to talk his way past the turnstiles. My uncle's basic strategy is to just keep moving. When he's greeted at the front desk, my uncle immediately asks for a towel, then exploits the confusion.

There are also successful variations of the two-in, one-out method. This tactic is modeled after the fraternity approach to college football games. Two people enter a stadium with legitimate passes; one person stays, while the other walks back out with two passes in his pocket, ready to retrieve someone from the outside. Here's how this works at the gym. You'll first check in at the front desk, then loudly forget something in your car. You give your card to your relative waiting outside, and stride back through with nothing, having already shown your bona fides.

Of course, there's always a chance that the front desk will be empty. Or better yet, the attendant simply doesn't care.

Yesterday, my mother and I drove to my gym with only my valid gym card and a local resident guest pass - totally inapplicable in her case. During the ride over, we rehearsed all kinds of stories and contingencies to get her through the gate.

At the turnstile, I scanned my card and she strolled through. I scanned my card again and I strolled through. We both nodded to the woman behind the desk and headed toward the locker rooms.

Just keep moving.

## A Universal Top 10 List

I've written a lot about why people don't want to go to the gym. Now, I thought it might be interesting to focus on why people do.

I came across an announcement that made headlines across the country, the results of a recent study about people's motivation to have sex. Though you'd assume people have sex for simple and straightforward reasons, the research revealed dozens of varied and complex motivations - 237 in all.

I've inserted a chart below. The left side shows the top 10 most intriguing reasons people gave for having sex, and the right side shows the top 10 reasons I think people are motivated to go to the gym.

| TOP 10 REASONS FOR HAVING SEX | TOP 10 REASONS FOR GOING TO THE GYM |
|---|---|
| 1. I was sexually aroused and wanted the release | 1. I was sexually aroused and wanted the release |
| 2. I wanted to stop my partner's nagging | 2. I wanted to stop my partner's nagging |
| 3. I wanted to improve my sexual skills | 3. I wanted to improve my sexual skills |
| 4. I wanted to get a new job | 4. I wanted to get a new job |
| 5. I wanted to be popular | 5. I wanted to be popular |
| 6. I wanted to get rid of a headache | 6. I wanted to get rid of a headache |
| 7. I wanted to keep my partner from straying | 7. I wanted to keep my partner from straying |
| 8. I thought it would make me feel healthy | 8. I thought it would make me feel healthy |

9. I wanted to see what the
fuss is all about

9. I wanted to see what the fuss
is all about

10. I thought it would help me
to fall asleep

10. I thought it would help me
to fall asleep

## Door Man

A few years ago my gym closed the men's locker room for renovation, and during this time turned the women's locker room into a unisex bathroom. I don't remember how this played out exactly – I guess showering was reserved for only those without the least sense of modesty. I do recall thinking like a third-grade boy how cool it was to be hanging out in the women's bathroom, if only just to throw my gym bag into a locker. I also felt there was sure to be trouble when the men's room finally reopened, and guys still walked into the ladies' room out of force of habit.

I don't think it's possible to overstate the importance of an exterior locker room door. For example, my gym was able to cover the ladies' room door with warnings during and after renovation - one last deterrent against a co-gender calamity. At many gyms, however, the locker room entrances are nothing more than cavernous openings, with privacy achieved through the architecture of interior walls.

I recently worked out at a gym I hadn't visited in a number of years. The entire gym had been overhauled, and the locker rooms were completely redone. For whatever reason, the location of the men's and women's locker rooms had also been reversed. Only a small sign on the wall by each opening indicated which members belonged where.

Just like old times, I powered through a tough workout at this gym. I finished exercising and wandered into the men's room, my head down in a post-workout fog.

When I looked up, I was surprised not only by how substantially the layout of the men's room had changed in the last hour, but also by the presence of two women wearing only shorts and bras. I suddenly realized I had two choices. I could either say "Oops, sorry!" and sprint out of there, clearing my conscience but drawing attention to myself. Or, I could quietly reverse course and slip away like some peeping-tom. While I debated these choices in my head, my legs took over. I spun away from my blunder and rushed out, diving into the sanctuary of the adjacent men's room.

## Why in Deed

Anyone who makes exercise a regular part of his or her routine has to acknowledge Jerry Seinfeld's point about the circular logic of the gym:

> "The only reason that you're getting in shape is so you can get through the workout. So we're working out, so that we'll be in shape, for when we have to do our exercises."

I'll pile on even a bit more, questioning exercise's supposed ability to make you "feel better." The day after I train legs, an ordinary flight of stairs looks to me more like a mountain. Depending upon what's happening with my low back, tying my shoes can be a real struggle. And I'm hard pressed to see the advantage of using up your energy for the day prior to 7 a.m.

So truly, why bother?

Well, upon further reflection, I've compiled a list of times when I've found the effort to stay fit - and a thick layer of muscle - to actually come in handy:

10. Getting off the subway: You're sitting in the center of the metro car as the train pulls into your station; you count about 30 people - plus assorted luggage, instrument cases and bicycles - standing between you and the door, which will remain open for only a matter of seconds.

9. Protecting your internal organs: When you're resting on your bed, and your kids start to use your torso as a trampoline, you can giggle right along with them.

8. Getting on the subway: You want to board an already packed subway train; as the door opens, you apply the gentle but firm encouragement of your forearm into the middle backs of the folks in front of you.

7. Eating contest: Due to your continual craving for food, you can impress friends and relatives with your ability to consume large quantities in a short period of time. (Downside: constant hunger can also get expensive.)

6. Trying to catch an early flight: At the bus stop, you figure out the hard way that bus service to the metro doesn't start for another hour; it's no problem for you to walk instead, making the one mile trek up to the train station while dragging along your bulging suitcase.

5. Feats of strength: When your massive picture tube television finally dies, you can haul it out to the curb solo, without needing to call in a favor from friends or neighbors.

4. Saving time: It only takes one trip to carry all the grocery bags in your car up the stairs and into the kitchen.

3. Crash recovery: When you lace up ice skates for the first time in 20 years, you can survive the inevitable wipeout without serious trauma.

2. Discipline: When you inform your uncooperative children they have the opportunity to complete a task (i.e., getting dressed, going upstairs) "the easy way or the hard way," you can, when necessary, make good on the threat.

1. Shoveling snow: When the forecast calls for snow, you don't need to worry about the aftermath causing heart trouble or other injury. In fact, if snow has made the roads impassable, the shoveling can substitute for your trip to the gym.

**Honey vs. Vinegar**

It's been a while since I've been scolded by gym staff for dropping my heavy dumbbells at the end of a set. Not only do I try my best to treat gym equipment with care, but most gyms have also upgraded to rubber-encased dumbbells. Iron missiles now impact resilient, high-tech floors with barely a thud.

Still, gym staff trying to look busy can always shuffle over to the dumbbell rack and hassle someone training hard.

Over the past few years, the fierce competition among gyms has perhaps caused the demeanor of gym staff to improve; or possibly, the modern gym's high ceilings and bright colors have softened the typical employee's disposition. Either way, I have to say that the reprimand I got this morning almost made my day: "Hey there – yes you – you need to be more careful about dropping your weights ... otherwise, I was very impressed."

**Time Machine**

Waiting for a meeting to start, a younger colleague of mine began filling the air with a story about her previous night's fun. With the conference room falling silent, someone blurted out: "We all have 23 year-old envy!"

Well, I'm not so sure. The Internet is awash in articles with titles like: Things I Wish I Could Tell My Younger Self About Dating/Careers/Money. In fact, it seems that what people really want is to go back in time and shake their younger selves by the lapel. So, given the chance, here are five things about exercise I'd shout into the ear of my 23 year-old self.

5) Learn how to jump rope. Yes, you can pick up the jump rope in your 30s, but the coordination is easier to learn at a younger age, and advanced moves can take years to perfect. Besides, the fitness you build jumping rope strengthens every part of your routine, making you a faster runner and a more powerful lifter. Enjoy the benefits as soon as possible.

4) Squat correctly. I know that when you started lifting, you used to squat with a block of wood under your heels. Maybe you've learned by now to squat only with your heels planted firmly on the floor. In any event, I have finally started to squat correctly, with my feet spread wide and my knees thrust out. My knees no longer hurt, my hamstrings are huge, and I haven't thrown out my back in over a year. Speaking of throwing out our back …

3) You only have one low back. Now, all those sets of Good Mornings, I understand. Gyms used to post pictures of Good Mornings as a recommended back exercise until angry mobs started tearing them down. Regardless, the 345 pound deadlifts were just dumb. We even got in trouble for all the noise we were making (see Chapter 4).

2) Pick a weight that causes you to fail at 10 reps. Anything heavier than that and you're setting yourself up for injury. It doesn't matter how heavy you can go on a particular day if you can't make it back in for a week, or longer.

1) Stop doing upright rows. I read an article several years ago about how the top of the movement causes fragile shoulder parts to squeeze and rub against each other. I replaced upright rows in my routine with raises of various kinds, and I've noticed no difference in shoulder strength or size.

Bonus tip: Cut the wheat out of your diet. Whether or not you believe in the paleo lifestyle, the bowls of multigrain cereal and stacks of whole wheat bagels just make it harder for you to show off all your great ab work.

# ABOUT THE AUTHOR

Keva Silversmith has been a fitness fanatic for his entire adult life, with the war stories and chronic injuries to show for it. Keva has held an ACE personal training certification, experiencing the fitness industry from the inside and out.

Keva works currently as a public relations professional in Miami, Florida. He holds a J.D. from the University of Virginia and an M.A. in Speech Communications from Emerson College. Keva graduated from the University of Michigan with a B.A. in History.